The Indispensable Guide to Good Laboratory Practice (GLP)

Second Edition

Mark Gregory Slomiany Ph.D.

Pinehurst Press, Inc.
New York, NY

Table of Contents

Chapter 1

Introduction to GLP

1.01: What's GLP? Can I be Certified?

At its most basic, Good Laboratory Practice (GLP) provides the framework for how to conduct a stage 2 preclinical study if one is intending to submit an application to the FDA for research or marketing permits for products regulated by the FDA [for example, the submission of a new drug application (NDA)]. GLP covers topics like who coordinates the study, who does the study, how are the materials, animals, and facilities maintained, how is the data organized and stored, how are the report written, who checks the report, and what federal inspectors are looking for before and after the study is submitted to the FDA.

It should be noted that there is no such thing as an official certification in GLP. Sure you can demonstrate your knowledge of GLP by completing a training course or workshop, but you can equally demonstrate your understanding of GLP by reading up on the subject and having a grasp on the key concepts and their application. As such, this guide was written to breathe a bit of life into the dusty list of GLP regulations, providing an understanding of not only what they are, but how the components fit together in conducting an FDA compliant non-clinical laboratory study.

1.02 The GLP Framwork

GLPs are guidelines set forth by the FDA to regulate the process of conducting non-clinical laboratory studies intended to support applications for research or marketing permits for products regulated by the FDA, or by similar other national agencies. This includes non-clinical safety studies of development of drugs, biological products, and medical devices, as well as agricultural pesticide development, development of toxic chemicals, food control (food additives), and tests of substances with regard to explosive hazards.

Good Laboratory Practice (GLP) deals with the *organization*, *process* and *conditions* under which laboratory studies are conducted. They are intended to promote not only the *quality*, but the *validity* of test data as well. Consequently, GLP regulations and guidelines have a significant impact on the daily operation of an analytical laboratory, influencing 5 key areas of the experimental process:

1. planning
2. performing
3. monitoring
4. recording
5. reporting

Beyond good analytical practice, GLP is a regulation. Indeed, though good analytical practice is important, it is not enough. For example, the laboratory must have a specific organizational structure and procedures to perform and document laboratory work. Thus, the objective is not only quality of data but also traceability and integrity of data, whether it be immediately after the study has been finished or even 5 or 10 years henceforth. As such, GLP provides a standard methodology whereby a GLP inspector can examine documentation and easily find out:

-Who has done a study?

-How was the experiment was carried out?

-Which procedures have been used?

-Were there any problems?

-If there were any problems, how were they solved?

Thus, in its most basic sense, GLP can be broken down into five rather logical requirements:

1. Responsibilities should be defined for the:
    - Sponsor management
    - Study management
    - Quality assurance unit
2. All routine work should follow written standard operating procedures.
3. Facilities such as laboratories should be large enough and be constructed correctly to ensure the integrity of a study
3. Test and control articles should have the right quality and instruments should be calibrated and well maintained
4. People should be trained or otherwise qualified for the job
5. Raw data and other data should be acquired, processed and archived to ensure integrity of data.

1.03: When do I use GLP? What about GCP or GMP?

Drug development can be divided into a number of stages. However, note that only stage 2 involves GLP regulatory standards:

STAGE 1

The first stage, the discovery of potential new drug products, is not covered by a regulatory standard, nor are studies demonstrating proof of concept. This area may well require some international standards or guidance documents in the future.

STAGE 2

Toxicology and safety pharmacology studies, with a potential extension to pharmacokinetics and bioavailability require compliance with GLP. These studies are termed "non-clinical" as they are not performed in humans. Their primary purpose is safety testing.

STAGE 3

The third stage, following on from safety studies, encompasses the clinical studies in human. Here, good clinical practice (GCP) is the basis for quality standards, ethical conduct and regulatory compliance. GCP must be instituted in all clinical trials from Phase I (to demonstrate tolerance of the test drug and to define human pharmacokinetics), through Phase II (where the dose-effect relationship is confirmed), to Phase III (full-scale, often multicentre, clinical efficacy trials in hundreds of patients). From stage 3 of development and continuing throughout the rest of the drug's lifetime, good manufacturing practice (GMP) applies to all manufacturing of bulk and formulated product.

STAGE 4

The fourth stage is post-approval. Here the drug is registered and available on the market. However, even after marketing, the use of the drug is monitored through formalized pharmacovigilance procedures3. Any subsequent clinical trials (Phase IV) must also comply with GCP.

1.04: GLP Summary: *When you need it and when you don't*

Typically, basic research, disease discovery, and drug discovery is NOT regulated. GLP only starts with preclinical development, for example toxicology studies. Clinical trials (stage 1-4) are regulated by GCP regulations and manufacturing regulations through GMPs. There is a frequent misunderstanding that all laboratory operations are regulated by GLP. This isn't so! For example, Quality Control laboratories in manufacturing are regulated by GMPs and not by GLPs. Furthermore, Good Laboratory Practice regulations are frequently mixed up with good analytical practice. Applying good analytical practices is important but not sufficient.

In other words, GLPs regulate all non-clinical safety studies that support or are intended to support applications for research or marketing permits for products regulated by the FDA, or by similar other national agencies. This includes non-clinical safety studies of development of drugs, biological products, and medical devices, as well as agricultural pesticide development, development of toxic chemicals, food control (food additives), and tests of substances with regard to explosive hazards. *The duration and location of the study is inconsequential.* Conversely, basic research, studies to develop new analytical methods, and chemical tests used to derive the specifications of a marketed food product are NOT covered.

1.05: A Brief History on the Evolution of GLP

The formal concept of 'good laboratory practice' first evolved in the USA in the 1970s due to concerns about the validity of preclinical safety data submitted to the Food and Drug Administration (FDA) in the context of new drug applications (NDA). The inspection of studies and test facilities had yielded indications for, and instances of, inadequate planning and incompetent execution of studies, insufficient documentation of methods and results, and even fraud. For example, replacing animals which died during a study by new ones; deleting necropsy observations because the histopathologist received no specimens of lesions; or re-correcting discrepancies in raw data and final report tables by juggling around the raw data in order to 'fit the results tables' to the final report. These deficiencies were made public in the so-called Kennedy Hearings of the US Congress, and the political outcome of these subsequently led to the publication, by the FDA, of Proposed Regulations on GLP in 1976, with the respective Final Rule coming into effect in June 1979 (21 CFR 58). These regulations were intended to provide the regulatory basis for assurance that reports on studies submitted to the FDA would reflect faithfully and completely the experimental work carried out. It should be noted that in the chemical and pesticide field, the US Environmental Protection Agency (EPA) had encountered similar problems with study quality and issued its own draft GLP regulations in 1979 and 1980, publishing the Final Rules in two separate parts (40 CFR 160 and 40 CFR 792, reflecting the different legal bases) in 1983.

1.06: How do I use this book?

The FDA describes GLP or officially "Good Laboratory Practice for Nonclinical Laboratory Studies" in Title 21, Part 58 of the Code of Federal Regulations. As detailed in the next section, they divide it into subparts (A-K), with each subpart describing an aspect of GLP. As such, each chapter of this book will cover one of these subparts. However, rather than abandoning you to the torture of FDA legalese, I have attempted to summarize each section in the introduction to each chapter. Through reading these summaries, you will not only learn about the regulations, but the structure and key players of a GLP laboratory and how they interact. If you still want to learn more or are just plain fighting insomnia, then continue to the official FDA verbiage provided below each chapter summary.

1.07: Layout of Title 21, Part 58 "Good Laboratory Practice for Nonclinical Laboratory Studies (*subparts A-K*)

Subpart A--General Provisions

§ 58.1 - Scope.

§ 58.3 - Definitions.

§ 58.10 - Applicability to studies performed under grants and contracts.

§ 58.15 - Inspection of a testing facility.

Subpart B--Organization and Personnel

§ 58.29 - Personnel.

§ 58.31 - Testing facility management.

§ 58.33 - Study director.

§ 58.35 - Quality assurance unit.

Subpart C--Facilities

§ 58.41 - General.

§ 58.43 - Animal care facilities.

§ 58.45 - Animal supply facilities.

§ 58.47 - Facilities for handling test and control articles.

§ 58.49 - Laboratory operation areas.

§ 58.51 - Specimen and data storage facilities.

Subpart D--Equipment

§ 58.61 - Equipment design.

§ 58.63 - Maintenance and calibration of equipment.

Subpart E--Testing Facilities Operation

§ 58.81 - Standard operating procedures.

§ 58.83 - Reagents and solutions.

§ 58.90 - Animal care.

Authority: 21 U.S.C. 342, 346, 346a, 348, 351, 352, 353, 355, 360, 360b-360f, 360h-360j, 371, 379e, 381; 42 U.S.C. 216, 262, 263b-263n.

Source: 43 FR 60013, Dec. 22, 1978, unless otherwise noted.

CHAPTER 2

Subpart A—General Provisions

58.1 Scope

58.3 Definitions

58.10 Applicability to studies performed under grants and contracts

58.15 Inspection of a testing facility

Summary

58.1 Scope- The scope defines the kind of studies covered by the principles of GLP. Namely, that they should be applied to the non-clinical safety testing of test items contained in pharmaceutical products, pesticide products, cosmetic products, veterinary drugs as well as food additives, feed additives, and industrial chemicals. These test items are frequently synthetic chemicals, but may be of natural or biological origin and, in some circumstances, may be living organisms.

58.3 Definitions- The definition of terms contained in these subparts.

58.10 Applicability to studies performed under grants and contracts- When you're conducting a nonclinical laboratory study intended to be submitted to or reviewed by the Food and Drug Administration and contract out for these testing services, you need to notify the contractor that the study has to be conducted in compliance with GLP.

58.15 Inspection of a testing facility- Your testing facility has to let the FDA inspect the facility, records, and specimens that are required to be maintained under GLP guidelines. If you don't, then your application to the FDA will not be considered. However, even if your application is disqualified, that doesn't relieve you of the obligation to submit the results of the study to the FDA if required.

REGULATIONS: Subpart A—General Provisions

Sec. 58.1 Scope.

A. This part prescribes good laboratory practices for conducting nonclinical laboratory studies that support or are intended to support applications for research or marketing permits for products regulated by the Food and Drug Administration, including food and color additives, animal food additives, human and animal drugs, medical devices for human use, biological products, and electronic products. Compliance with this part is intended to assure the quality and integrity of the safety data filed pursuant to sections 406, 408, 409, 502, 503, 505, 506, 510, 512-516, 518-520, 721, and 801 of the Federal Food, Drug, and Cosmetic Act and sections 351 and 354-360F of the Public Health Service Act.

B. References in this part to regulatory sections of the Code of Federal Regulations are to chapter I of title 21, unless otherwise noted.

[43 FR 60013, Dec. 22, 1978, as amended at 52 FR 33779, Sept. 4, 1987; 64 FR 399, Jan. 5, 1999]

Sec. 58.3 Definitions.

As used in this part, the following terms shall have the meanings specified:

A. Act means the Federal Food, Drug, and Cosmetic Act, as amended (secs. 201-902, 52 Stat. 1040et seq., as amended (21 U.S.C. 321-392)).

B. Test article means any food additive, color additive, drug, biological product, electronic product, medical device for human use, or any other article subject to regulation under the act or under sections 351 and 354-360F of the Public Health Service Act.

C. Control article means any food additive, color additive, drug, biological product, electronic product, medical device for human use, or any article other than a test article, feed, or water that is administered to the test system in the course of a nonclinical laboratory study for the purpose of establishing a basis for comparison with the test article.

D. Nonclinical laboratory study means in vivo or in vitro experiments in which test articles are studied prospectively in test systems under laboratory conditions to determine their safety. The term does not include studies utilizing human subjects or clinical studies or field trials in animals. The term does not include basic exploratory studies carried out to determine whether a test article has any potential utility or to determine physical or chemical characteristics of a test article.

E. Application for research or marketing permit includes:
   1. A color additive petition, described in part 71.
   2. A food additive petition, described in parts 171 and 571.
   3. Data and information regarding a substance submitted as part of the procedures for establishing that a substance is generally recognized as safe for use, which use results or may reasonably be expected to result, directly or indirectly, in its becoming a component or otherwise affecting the characteristics of any food, described in 170.35 and 570.35.
   4. Data and information regarding a food additive submitted as part of the procedures regarding food additives permitted to be used on an interim basis pending additional study, described in 180.1.
   5. An investigational new drug application, described in part 312 of this chapter.
   6. Anew drug application, described in part 314.
   7. Data and information regarding an over-the-counter drug for human use, submitted as part of the procedures for classifying such drugs as generally recognized as safe and effective and not misbranded, described in part 330.

8. Data and information about a substance submitted as part of the procedures for establishing a tolerance for unavoidable contaminants in food and food-packaging materials, described in parts 109 and 509.

9. [Reserved]

10. ANotice of Claimed Investigational Exemption for a New Animal Drug, described in part 511.

11. Anew animal drug application, described in part 514.

12. [Reserved]

13. An application for a biologics license, described in part 601 of this chapter.

14. An application for an investigational device exemption, described in part 812.

15. An Application for Premarket Approval of a Medical Device, described in section 515 of the act.

16. A Product Development Protocol for a Medical Device, described in section 515 of the act.

17. Data and information regarding a medical device submitted as part of the procedures for classifying such devices, described in part 860.

18. Data and information regarding a medical device submitted as part of the procedures for establishing, amending, or repealing a performance standard for such devices, described in part 861.

19. Data and information regarding an electronic product submitted as part of the procedures for obtaining an exemption from notification of a radiation safety defect or failure of compliance with a radiation safety performance standard, described in subpart D of part 1003.

20. Data and information regarding an electronic product submitted as part of the procedures for establishing, amending, or repealing a standard for such product, described in section 358 of the Public Health Service Act.

21. Data and information regarding an electronic product submitted as part of the procedures for obtaining a variance from any electronic product performance standard as described in 1010.4.

22. Data and information regarding an electronic product submitted as part of the procedures for granting, amending, or extending an exemption from any electronic product performance standard, as described in 1010.5.
23. A premarket notification for a food contact substance, described in part 170, subpart D, of this chapter.

F. Sponsor means:
1. A person who initiates and supports, by provision of financial or other resources, a nonclinical laboratory study;
2. A person who submits a nonclinical study to the Food and Drug Administration in support of an application for a research or marketing permit; or
3. A testing facility, if it both initiates and actually conducts the study.

G. Testing facility means a person who actually conducts a nonclinical laboratory study, i.e., actually uses the test article in a test system. Testing facility includes any establishment required to register under section 510 of the act that conducts nonclinical laboratory studies and any consulting laboratory described in section 704 of the act that conducts such studies. Testing facility encompasses only those operational units that are being or have been used to conduct nonclinical laboratory studies.

H. Person includes an individual, partnership, corporation, association, scientific or academic establishment, government agency, or organizational unit thereof, and any other legal entity.

I. Test system means any animal, plant, microorganism, or subparts thereof to which the test or control article is administered or added for study. Test system also includes appropriate groups or components of the system not treated with the test or control articles.

J. Specimen means any material derived from a test system for examination or analysis.

K. Raw data means any laboratory worksheets, records, memoranda, notes, or exact copies thereof, that are the result of original observations and activities of a nonclinical laboratory study and are necessary for the reconstruction and evaluation of the report of that study. In the event that exact transcripts of raw data have been prepared (e.g., tapes which have been transcribed verbatim, dated, and verified accurate by signature), the exact copy or exact transcript may be substituted for the original source as raw data. Raw data may include photographs, microfilm or microfiche copies, computer printouts, magnetic media, including dictated observations, and recorded data from automated instruments.

L. Quality assurance unit means any person or organizational element, except the study director, designated by testing facility management to perform the duties relating to quality assurance of nonclinical laboratory studies.

M. Study director means the individual responsible for the overall conduct of a nonclinical laboratory study.

N. Batch means a specific quantity or lot of a test or control article that has been characterized according to 58.105(a).

O. Study initiation date means the date the protocol is signed by the study director.

P. Study completion date means the date the final report is signed by the study director.

[43 FR 60013, Dec. 22, 1978, as amended at 52 FR 33779, Sept. 4, 1987; 54 FR 9039, Mar. 3, 1989; 64 FR 56448, Oct. 20, 1999; 67 FR 35729, May 21, 2002]

Sec. 58.10 Applicability to studies performed under grants and contracts.

When a sponsor conducting a nonclinical laboratory study intended to be submitted to or reviewed by the Food and Drug Administration utilizes the services of a consulting laboratory, contractor, or grantee to perform an analysis or other service, it shall notify the consulting laboratory, contractor, or grantee that the service is part of a nonclinical laboratory study that must be conducted in compliance with the provisions of this part.

Sec. 58.15 Inspection of a testing facility.

A. A testing facility shall permit an authorized employee of the Food and Drug Administration, at reasonable times and in a reasonable manner, to inspect the facility and to inspect (and in the case of records also to copy) all records and specimens required to be maintained regarding studies within the scope of this part. The records inspection and copying requirements shall not apply to quality assurance unit records of findings and problems, or to actions recommended and taken.

B. The Food and Drug Administration will not consider a nonclinical laboratory study in support of an application for a research or marketing permit if the testing facility refuses to permit inspection. The determination that a nonclinical laboratory study will not be considered in support of an application for a research or marketing permit does not, however, relieve the applicant for such a permit of any obligation under any applicable statute or regulation to submit the results of the study to the Food and Drug Administration.

Authority: 21 U.S.C. 342, 346, 346a, 348, 351, 352, 353, 355, 360, 360b-360f, 360h-360j, 371, 379e, 381; 42 U.S.C. 216, 262, 263b-263n.
Source: 43 FR 60013, Dec. 22, 1978, unless otherwise noted.

CHAPTER 3

Subpart B—Organization and Personnel

58.29   Personnel.

58.31   Testing facility management.

58.33   Study director.

58.35   Quality assurance unit.

Summary

<u>58.29 Personnel</u>- The FDA insists that you have a sufficient number of qualified people to conduct GLP studies. They're not specific about the type of qualification or education, but whether the qualifications come from education, experience or additional trainings, it should be documented. Logically, this also requires a good documentation of the job descriptions, the tasks and responsibilities.

<u>58.31 Testing facility management</u>- The people coordinating the full portfolio of studies. They are responsible for appointing the 3 key players of a GLP study, namely:

1. **the study director**—the person who runs the study
2. **qualified personnel**—the underlings serving under the study director, conducting the GLP studies
3. **the quality assurance unit**—the in-house monitors required to check up on the study and give regular reports on the study's compliance to GLP

Basically, the buck stops with facility management. They designate a **study director** and consequently monitor the progress of the study. If it is not going well, it is up to them to replace the study director. Among other things, they should assure that a **quality assurance unit** is available, test and control articles are characterized, and that sufficient **qualified personnel** is available for the study. This is a back and forth interplay as obviously management can't be everywhere at once. So they rely on these groups to report to them. For example, GLPs require that the QA should give a regular report on the compliance status of the study.

<u>58.33 Study Director</u>—The position of a study director is unique for GLP. He/she has overall responsibility for the technical conduct of the safety studies, as well as for the

interpretation, analysis, documentation and reporting of the results. Designated by and supported by management, the study director serves as the single point of study control. It is important that this is a single individual person and not a department or any other grouping of people. An assistant study director is not permitted but there may be an alternate study director who serves as study director only in that person's absence. The study director may be the laboratory manager and may be responsible for more than one study. However, he/she should not be over-burdened—an auditor could otherwise get the impression that the study director cannot monitor all studies carefully.

58.35 Quality assurance unit (QAU)—The QAU serves an internal control function, responsible for monitoring each study to assure management that facilities, equipment, personnel, methods, practices, records, controls, standard operating procedures (SOPs), final reports (for data integrity), and archives are in conformance with the GLP/GALP regulations. Basically they're around to prevent nasty surprises when the FDA or EPA inspector comes to visit or after the study is submitted. Naturally, to prevent conflicts of interest, the QAU of a study is entirely separate and independent from the personnel engaged in the direction and conduct of the study to be monitored. Beyond immediately reporting any problems or issues, the QAU must maintain and periodically submit to laboratory management comprehensive written records listing findings and problems, actions recommended and taken, and scheduled dates for inspection. A representative from the FDA or EPA may ask to see the written procedures established for the QAU's inspection and may request the laboratory's management to certify that inspections are being implemented, and followed-up in accordance with the regulations governing the QAU. Full-time professionals are preferred over part-timers, because such an arrangement provides a degree of independence and removes the possibility that the demands of the person's second job will interfere with his or her performance of the QA function. The FDA mandates that responsibilities and procedures applicable to the QAU, the records maintained by the QAU, and the method of indexing such records be in writing and be maintained. The agency further requires that these items, including inspection dates, the description of the study inspected, the phase or segment of the study, and the name of the individual performing the inspection, be made available for review by an authorized FDA agent. The FDA agent cannot request the findings of the QAU audit .

QAU Responsibilities include:

1. Maintain a copy of master schedule sheet of all studies conducted. These are to be indexed by test article and must contain the test system, nature of study, date the study was initiated, current status of each study, identity of the sponsor, and name of the study director.

2. Maintain copies of all protocols pertaining to the studies for which QAU is responsible.

3. Inspect studies at intervals adequate to assure the integrity of the study and maintain written and properly signed records of each periodic inspection. These records must show the date of the inspection, the study inspected, the phase or segment of the study inspected, the person performing the inspection, findings and problems, action recommended and taken to resolve existing problems, and any scheduled date for re-inspection. Any problems discovered which are likely to affect study integrity are to be brought to the attention of the study director and management immediately.

4. Periodically submit to management and the study director written status reports on each study, noting problems and corrective actions taken.

5. Determine whether deviations from protocols and SOPs were made with proper authorization and documentation.

6. Review the final study report to assure that it accurately describes the methods and SOPs and that the reported results accurately reflect the raw data of the study.

7. Prepare and sign a statement to be included with the final study report that specifies the dates of audits and dates of reports to management and to the study director.

8. Audit the correctness of the statement, made by the study director, on the GLP compliance of the study.

REGULATIONS: Subpart B—Organization and Personnel

Sec. 58.29 Personnel.

A. Each individual engaged in the conduct of or responsible for the supervision of a nonclinical laboratory study shall have education, training, and experience, or combination thereof, to enable that individual to perform the assigned functions.

B. Each testing facility shall maintain a current summary of training and experience and job description for each individual engaged in or supervising the conduct of a nonclinical laboratory study.

C. There shall be a sufficient number of personnel for the timely and proper conduct of the study according to the protocol.

D. Personnel shall take necessary personal sanitation and health precautions designed to avoid contamination of test and control articles and test systems.

E. Personnel engaged in a nonclinical laboratory study shall wear clothing appropriate for the duties they perform. Such clothing shall be changed as often as necessary to prevent microbiological, radiological, or chemical contamination of test systems and test and control articles.

F. Any individual found at any time to have an illness that may adversely affect the quality and integrity of the nonclinical laboratory study shall be excluded from direct contact with test systems, test and control articles and any other operation or function that may adversely affect the study until the condition is corrected. All personnel shall be instructed to report to their immediate supervisors any health or medical conditions that may reasonably be considered to have an adverse effect on a nonclinical laboratory study.

Sec. 58.31 Testing facility management.

For each nonclinical laboratory study, testing facility management shall:

A. Designate a study director as described in 58.33, before the study is initiated.

B. Replace the study director promptly if it becomes necessary to do so during the conduct of a study.

C. Assure that there is a quality assurance unit as described in 58.35.

D. Assure that test and control articles or mixtures have been appropriately tested for identity, strength, purity, stability, and uniformity, as applicable.

E. Assure that personnel, resources, facilities, equipment, materials, and methodologies are available as scheduled.

F. Assure that personnel clearly understand the functions they are to perform.

G. Assure that any deviations from these regulations reported by the quality assurance unit are communicated to the study director and corrective actions are taken and documented.

[43 FR 60013, Dec. 22, 1978, as amended at 52 FR 33780, Sept. 4, 1987]

Sec. 58.33 Study director.

For each nonclinical laboratory study, a scientist or other professional of appropriate education, training, and experience, or combination thereof, shall be identified as the study director. The study director has overall responsibility for the technical conduct of the study, as well as for the interpretation, analysis, documentation and reporting of results, and represents the single point of study control. The study director shall assure that:

A. The protocol, including any change, is approved as provided by 58.120 and is followed.

B. All experimental data, including observations of unanticipated responses of the test system are accurately recorded and verified.

C. Unforeseen circumstances that may affect the quality and integrity of the nonclinical laboratory study are noted when they occur, and corrective action is taken and documented.

D. Test systems are as specified in the protocol.

E. All applicable good laboratory practice regulations are followed.

F. All raw data, documentation, protocols, specimens, and final reports are transferred to the archives during or at the close of the study.

[43 FR 60013, Dec. 22, 1978; 44 FR 17657, Mar. 23, 1979]

Sec. 58.35 Quality assurance unit.

A. A testing facility shall have a quality assurance unit which shall be responsible for monitoring each study to assure management that the facilities, equipment, personnel, methods, practices, records, and controls are in conformance with the regulations in this part. For any given study, the quality assurance unit shall be entirely separate from and independent of the personnel engaged in the direction and conduct of that study.

B. The quality assurance unit shall:

1. Maintain a copy of a master schedule sheet of all nonclinical laboratory studies conducted at the testing facility indexed by test article and containing the test system, nature of study, date study was initiated, current status of each study, identity of the sponsor, and name of the study director.

2. Maintain copies of all protocols pertaining to all nonclinical laboratory studies for which the unit is responsible.

3. Inspect each nonclinical laboratory study at intervals adequate to assure the integrity of the study and maintain written and properly signed records of each periodic inspection showing the date of the inspection, the study inspected, the phase or segment of the study inspected, the person performing the inspection, findings and problems, action recommended and taken to resolve existing problems, and any scheduled date for reinspection. Any problems found during the course of an inspection which are likely to affect study integrity shall be brought to the attention of the study director and management immediately.

4. Periodically submit to management and the study director written status reports on each study, noting any problems and the corrective actions taken.

5. Determine that no deviations from approved protocols or standard operating procedures were made without proper authorization and documentation.

6. Review the final study report to assure that such report accurately describes the methods and standard operating procedures, and that the reported results accurately reflect the raw data of the nonclinical laboratory study.

7. Prepare and sign a statement to be included with the final study report which shall specify the dates inspections were made and findings reported to management and to the study director.

C. The responsibilities and procedures applicable to the quality assurance unit, the records maintained by the quality assurance unit, and the method of indexing such records shall be in writing and shall be maintained. These items including inspection dates, the study inspected, the phase or segment of the study inspected, and the name of the individual performing the inspection shall be made available for inspection to authorized employees of the Food and Drug Administration.

D. A designated representative of the Food and Drug Administration shall have access to the written procedures established for the inspection and may request testing facility management to certify that inspections are being implemented, performed, documented, and followed-up in accordance with this paragraph.

[43 FR 60013, Dec. 22, 1978, as amended at 52 FR 33780, Sept. 4, 1987; 67 FR 9585, Mar. 4, 2002]

Authority: 21 U.S.C. 342, 346, 346a, 348, 351, 352, 353, 355, 360, 360b-360f, 360h-360j, 371, 379e, 381; 42 U.S.C. 216, 262, 263b-263n.
Source: 43 FR 60013, Dec. 22, 1978, unless otherwise noted.

CHAPTER 4

Subpart C—Facilities

58.41   **General.**

58.43   **Animal care facilities.**

58.45   **Animal supply facilities.**

58.47   **Facilities for handling test and control articles.**

58.49   **Laboratory operation areas.**

58.51   **Specimen and data storage facilities.**

<u>Summary</u>

<u>58.41 General</u>—The main purpose of these regulations are to ensure the integrity of the study and subsequent study data. Basically, there needs to be **limited access to the buildings and rooms, the facilities need to be large enough to comfortable run the study, and the study must be conducted in a facility that is designed to handle the work at hand.** For example, if the air handling is improperly configured, there may be cross contamination between different area. Or if there's a hole in the ceiling, the data will get wet when it rains.

<u>58.43 Animal care facilities</u>—If you use animals, there are regulations for keeping them healthy and happy.

<u>58.45 Animal supply facilities</u>—If you use animals, there are regulations for how to keep the food and bedding to keep your animals healthy and happy.

<u>58.47 Facilities for handling test and control articles</u>—You need separate facilities equipped with proper environmental and human error controls to prevent mixups and to keep your test and/or control substance/articles from going bad.

<u>58.49 Laboratory operation areas</u>—You need separate/dedicated laboratory space to do your nonclinical laboratory studies in.

<u>58.51 Specimen and data storage facilities</u>—You need dedicated space with limited access and proper environmental controls for the storage and retrieval of raw data and the specimens from completed studies.

REGULATIONS: Subpart C- Facilities

Sec. 58.41 General.

Each testing facility shall be of suitable size and construction to facilitate the proper conduct of nonclinical laboratory studies. It shall be designed so that there is a degree of separation that will prevent any function or activity from having an adverse effect on the study.

[52 FR 33780, Sept. 4, 1987]

Sec. 58.43 Animal care facilities.

A. A testing facility shall have a sufficient number of animal rooms or areas, as needed, to assure proper: (1) Separation of species or test systems, (2) isolation of individual projects, (3) quarantine of animals, and (4) routine or specialized housing of animals.

B. A testing facility shall have a number of animal rooms or areas separate from those described in paragraph (a) of this section to ensure isolation of studies being done with test systems or test and control articles known to be biohazardous, including volatile substances, aerosols, radioactive materials, and infectious agents.

C. Separate areas shall be provided, as appropriate, for the diagnosis, treatment, and control of laboratory animal diseases. These areas shall provide effective isolation for the housing of animals either known or suspected of being diseased, or of being carriers of disease, from other animals.

D. When animals are housed, facilities shall exist for the collection and disposal of all animal waste and refuse or for safe sanitary storage of waste before removal from the testing facility. Disposal facilities shall be so provided and operated as to minimize vermin infestation, odors, disease hazards, and environmental contamination.

[43 FR 60013, Dec. 22, 1978, as amended at 52 FR 33780, Sept. 4, 1987]

Sec. 58.45 Animal supply facilities.

There shall be storage areas, as needed, for feed, bedding, supplies, and equipment. Storage areas for feed and bedding shall be separated from areas housing the test systems and shall be protected against infestation or contamination. Perishable supplies shall be preserved by appropriate means.

[43 FR 60013, Dec. 22, 1978, as amended at 52 FR 33780, Sept. 4, 1987]

Sec. 58.47 Facilities for handling test and control articles.

A. As necessary to prevent contamination or mixups, there shall be separate areas for:

> **1.** Receipt and storage of the test and control articles.
>
> **2.** Mixing of the test and control articles with a carrier, e.g., feed.
>
> **3.** Storage of the test and control article mixtures.

B. Storage areas for the test and/or control article and test and control mixtures shall be separate from areas housing the test systems and shall be adequate to preserve the identity, strength, purity, and stability of the articles and mixtures.

Sec. 58.49 Laboratory operation areas.

Separate laboratory space shall be provided, as needed, for the performance of the routine and specialized procedures required by nonclinical laboratory studies.

[52 FR 33780, Sept. 4, 1987]

Sec. 58.51 Specimen and data storage facilities.

Space shall be provided for archives, limited to access by authorized personnel only, for the storage and retrieval of all raw data and specimens from completed studies.

Authority: 21 U.S.C. 342, 346, 346a, 348, 351, 352, 353, 355, 360, 360b-360f, 360h-360j, 371, 379e, 381; 42 U.S.C. 216, 262, 263b-263n.
Source: 43 FR 60013, Dec. 22, 1978, unless otherwise noted.

CHAPTER 5

Subpart D—Equipment

58.61   Equipment design.

58.63   Maintenance and calibration of equipment.

Summary

58.61 Equipment design—Equipment used in generation, measurement, or assessment of data and equipment used for facility environmental control needs to be appropriately designed to function as directed in your protocols and needs to be suitably located for operation, inspection, cleaning, and maintenance. The equipment needs to undergo a validation process to ensure that it will consistently function as intended.

58.63 Maintenance and calibration of equipment—Equipment needs to be adequately inspected, cleaned, and maintained. Equipment used for generation, measurement, or assessment of data needs to be adequately tested, calibrated and/or standardized. These activities are frequently called qualification for equipment hardware and single modules and validation for software and complete systems. A laboratory needs to establish schedules for such operations based on manufacturer's recommendations and laboratory experience. Thus, the frequency for calibration, re-validation and testing (performance verification) depends on the instrument itself, the recommendations from manufacturers of equipment, laboratory experience, and the extent of use. As with other procedures in the GLP laboratory, written records need to be maintained of all inspections, maintenance, testing, calibrating and/or qualification / validation operations. These records, containing the date of operation, need to describe whether the maintenance operations followed written SOPs. In addition, written records need to be kept of non-routine repairs performed on equipment as a result of failure and malfunction. Such records shall document the nature of the defect, how and when the defect was discovered, and any remedial action taken in response to the defect. Written records may be in log books especially designed for that purpose. A log book should accompany the instrument when it is moved. Remedial action should include a review of effects on data generated before the defect was discovered. Such equipment records should be maintained as long as the data generated by the equipment.

REGULATIONS: Subpart D—Equipment

Sec. 58.61 Equipment design.

Equipment used in the generation, measurement, or assessment of data and equipment used for facility environmental control shall be of appropriate design and adequate capacity to function according to the protocol and shall be suitably located for operation, inspection, cleaning, and maintenance.

[52 FR 33780, Sept. 4, 1987]

Sec. 58.63 Maintenance and calibration of equipment.

A. Equipment shall be adequately inspected, cleaned, and maintained. Equipment used for the generation, measurement, or assessment of data shall be adequately tested, calibrated and/or standardized.

B. The written standard operating procedures required under 58.81(b)(11) shall set forth in sufficient detail the methods, materials, and schedules to be used in the routine inspection, cleaning, maintenance, testing, calibration, and/or standardization of equipment, and shall specify, when appropriate, remedial action to be taken in the event of failure or malfunction of equipment. The written standard operating procedures shall designate the person responsible for the performance of each operation.

C. Written records shall be maintained of all inspection, maintenance, testing, calibrating and/or standardizing operations. These records, containing the date of the operation, shall describe whether the maintenance operations were routine and followed the written standard operating procedures. Written records shall be kept of nonroutine repairs performed on equipment as a result of failure and malfunction. Such records shall document the nature of the defect, how and when the defect was discovered, and any remedial action taken in response to the defect.

[43 FR 60013, Dec. 22, 1978, as amended at 52 FR 33780, Sept. 4, 1987; 67 FR 9585, Mar. 4, 2002]

Authority: 21 U.S.C. 342, 346, 346a, 348, 351, 352, 353, 355, 360, 360b-360f, 360h-360j, 371, 379e, 381; 42 U.S.C. 216, 262, 263b-263n.

Source: 43 FR 60013, Dec. 22, 1978, unless otherwise noted.

CHAPTER 6

Subpart E—Testing facilities operation

58.81   Standard operating procedures.

58.83   Reagents and solutions.

58.90   Animal care.

Summary

58.81 Standard operating procedures (SOPs)—These are written procedures for a laboratories program. They define how to carry out protocol-specified activities. Most often they are written in a chronological listing of action steps. SOPs include:

- Routine inspection, cleaning, maintenance, testing, calibration and standardization of instruments
- Actions to be taken in response to equipment failure
- Analytical methods
- Definition of raw data
- Data handling, storage, and retrieval
- Health and safety precautions
- Receipt, identification, storage, mixing, and method sampling of test and control articles
- Record keeping, reporting, storage, and retrieval of data
- Coding of studies, handling of data, including the use of computerized data systems
- Operation of quality assurance personnel in performing and reporting study audits, inspections, and final study report reviews

It is suggested that SOPs be written in the laboratory and possibly by or at least reviewed by the instruments' operators. Furthermore, they should be written in a way that makes it easy for other members of the laboratory to use the instruments. It should be noted that *SOPs are often the weak point of an inspection.* Indeed, SOPs are frequently mentioned as sticking points in FDA warning letters, specifically that they are not available, adequate, or followed. This isn't to say that SOPs must always be followed.

Rather, GLPs allows a laboratory to deviate from SOPs when deviations are approved and documented.

58.83   Reagents and solutions—The quality of reagents and solutions is crucial in GLP studies. Thus, their purchasing and testing should be handled by a quality assurance program and the qualification of suppliers verified. Subsequently, all reagents and solutions in the laboratory need to be labeled to indicate identity, titer or concentration, storage requirements, and expiration date. Formal studies are not always required to justify assigned expiration dates. It is sufficient to assign expiration dates based on literature references and/or laboratory experience, so it may be sufficient to write "none" on extremely stable chemicals, such as sodium chloride. However, deteriorated or outdated reagents and solutions can not be used. Finally, you will need to label all containers accordingly if reagents and solutions used for non-GLP regulated work are stored in the same room as reagents for GLP-regulated studies.

58.90 Animal care—The health of animals is crucial in GLP studies. Thus, there should be SOPs for the housing, feeding, handling, and care of animals. Basically, when they arrive, they should be isolated and evaluated to prevent infection of the general animal population. Animals used in the study need to be healthy and great care should be given to ensure the quality of their food and bedding. Naturally, animals of different species are required to be segregated accordingly. In addition, pest control substances used should be documented or restricted altogether if known to interfere with the study at hand.

REGULATIONS: Subpart E—Testing facilities operation

Sec. 58.81 Standard operating procedures.

A. A testing facility shall have standard operating procedures in writing setting forth nonclinical laboratory study methods that management is satisfied are adequate to insure the quality and integrity of the data generated in the course of a study. All deviations in a study from standard operating procedures shall be authorized by the study director and shall be documented in the raw data. Significant changes in established standard operating procedures shall be properly authorized in writing by management.

B. Standard operating procedures shall be established for, but not limited to, the following:

1. Animal room preparation.

2. Animal care.

3. Receipt, identification, storage, handling, mixing, and method of sampling of the test and control articles.

4. Test system observations.

5. Laboratory tests.

6. Handling of animals found moribund or dead during study.

7. Necropsy of animals or postmortem examination of animals.

8. Collection and identification of specimens.

9. Histopathology.

10. Data handling, storage, and retrieval.

11. Maintenance and calibration of equipment.

12. Transfer, proper placement, and identification of animals.

C. Each laboratory area shall have immediately available laboratory manuals and standard operating procedures relative to the laboratory procedures being performed. Published literature may be used as a supplement to standard operating procedures.

D. A historical file of standard operating procedures, and all revisions thereof, including the dates of such revisions, shall be maintained.

[43 FR 60013, Dec. 22, 1978, as amended at 52 FR 33780, Sept. 4, 1987]

Sec. 58.83 Reagents and solutions.

All reagents and solutions in the laboratory areas shall be labeled to indicate identity, titer or concentration, storage requirements, and expiration date. Deteriorated or outdated reagents and solutions shall not be used.

Sec. 58.90 Animal care.

A. There shall be standard operating procedures for the housing, feeding, handling, and care of animals.

B. All newly received animals from outside sources shall be isolated and their health status shall be evaluated in accordance with acceptable veterinary medical practice.

C. At the initiation of a nonclinical laboratory study, animals shall be free of any disease or condition that might interfere with the purpose or conduct of the study. If, during the course of the study, the animals contract such a disease or condition, the diseased animals shall be isolated, if necessary. These animals may be treated for disease or signs of disease provided that such treatment does not interfere with the study. The diagnosis, authorizations of treatment, description of treatment, and each date of treatment shall be documented and shall be retained.

D. Warm-blooded animals, excluding suckling rodents, used in laboratory procedures that require manipulations and observations over an extended period of time or in studies that require the animals to be removed from and returned to their home cages for any reason (e.g., cage cleaning, treatment, etc.), shall receive appropriate identification. All information needed to specifically identify each animal within an animal-housing unit shall appear on the outside of that unit.

E. Animals of different species shall be housed in separate rooms when necessary. Animals of the same species, but used in different studies, should not ordinarily be housed in the same room when inadvertent exposure to control or test articles or animal mixup could affect the outcome of either study. If such mixed housing is necessary, adequate differentiation by space and identification shall be made.

F. Animal cages, racks and accessory equipment shall be cleaned and sanitized at appropriate intervals.

G. Feed and water used for the animals shall be analyzed periodically to ensure that contaminants known to be capable of interfering with the study and reasonably expected to be present in such feed or water are not present at levels above those specified in the protocol. Documentation of such analyses shall be maintained as raw data.

H. Bedding used in animal cages or pens shall not interfere with the purpose or conduct of the study and shall be changed as often as necessary to keep the animals dry and clean.

I. If any pest control materials are used, the use shall be documented. Cleaning and pest control materials that interfere with the study shall not be used.

[43 FR 60013, Dec. 22, 1978, as amended at 52 FR 33780, Sept. 4, 1987; 54 FR 15924, Apr. 20, 1989; 56 FR 32088, July 15, 1991; 67 FR 9585, Mar. 4, 2002]

Authority: 21 U.S.C. 342, 346, 346a, 348, 351, 352, 353, 355, 360, 360b-360f, 360h-360j, 371, 379e, 381; 42 U.S.C. 216, 262, 263b-263n.
Source: 43 FR 60013, Dec. 22, 1978, unless otherwise noted.

CHAPTER 7

Subpart F—Test and Control Articles

58.105 Test and control article characterization.

58.107 Test and control article handling.

58.113 Mixtures of articles with carriers.

Summary

58.105 Test and control article characterization—To review, "test article" refers to the substance being tested, while "control article" refers to the reference substance that is commonly used to calibrate the instrument. Thus, the accuracy of the reference substances also determines the accuracy of the analytical method. In other words, if the reference standard is off, the test will be off. This subsection deals with the testing and documentation of both of these to control for batch to batch variability. The identity, strength, purity, composition and other characteristics of the test and control articles should be determined for each batch and documented. Methods of synthesis, fabrication, or derivation of test and control articles should also be documented. Copies of this documentation must be stored with the study data and must be available for FDA inspection. In addition, the stability of each test or control article should be determined. This can be done either before study initiation, or simultaneously according to written SOPs which provide for periodic reanalysis of each batch. Each storage container for a test or control article should be labeled by name, chemical abstract number, or code number, batch number, expiration date, and, where appropriate, storage conditions necessary to maintain the identity, strength, purity and composition. Finally, for studies of more than 4 weeks' duration, reserve samples from each batch of test and control articles should be retained for the length of the study.

58.107 Test and control article handling—Procedures need to be in place for the handling of the test and control articles to ensure that there is proper storage, documentation of distribution, and minimal risk of contamination, deterioration, damage, or loss of identification.

58.113 Mixtures of articles with carriers—Lets start with a definition. Drug carriers are substances that serve as mechanisms to improve the delivery and the effectiveness of drugs. So when combining the test or control article with a carrier, you've added another variable that needs testing and documentation. Thus, for each test or control article that is mixed with a carrier, analysis is needed to determine the uniformity, concentration, and stability of test and control articles. This subsection also requires that if one or more of the components of the mixture has an expiration date, the earliest date needs to be shown on the container.

REGULATIONS: Subpart F—Test and Control Articles

Sec. 58.105 Test and control article characterization.

A. The identity, strength, purity, and composition or other characteristics which will appropriately define the test or control article shall be determined for each batch and shall be documented. Methods of synthesis, fabrication, or derivation of the test and control articles shall be documented by the sponsor or the testing facility. In those cases where marketed products are used as control articles, such products will be characterized by their labeling.

B. The stability of each test or control article shall be determined by the testing facility or by the sponsor either: (1) Before study initiation, or (2) concomitantly according to written standard operating procedures, which provide for periodic analysis of each batch.

C. Each storage container for a test or control article shall be labeled by name, chemical abstract number or code number, batch number, expiration date, if any, and, where appropriate, storage conditions necessary to maintain the identity, strength, purity, and composition of the test or control article. Storage containers shall be assigned to a particular test article for the duration of the study.

D. For studies of more than 4 weeks' duration, reserve samples from each batch of test and control articles shall be retained for the period of time provided by 58.195.

[43 FR 60013, Dec. 22, 1978, as amended at 52 FR 33781, Sept. 4, 1987; 67 FR 9585, Mar. 4, 2002]

Sec. 58.107 Test and control article handling.

Procedures shall be established for a system for the handling of the test and control articles to ensure that:

A. There is proper storage.

B. Distribution is made in a manner designed to preclude the possibility of contamination, deterioration, or damage.

C. Proper identification is maintained throughout the distribution process.

D. The receipt and distribution of each batch is documented. Such documentation shall include the date and quantity of each batch distributed or returned.

Sec. 58.113 Mixtures of articles with carriers.

A. For each test or control article that is mixed with a carrier, tests by appropriate analytical methods shall be conducted:

    1. To determine the uniformity of the mixture and to determine, periodically, the concentration of the test or control article in the mixture.

    2. To determine the stability of the test and control articles in the mixture as required by the conditions of the study either:

        i. Before study initiation, or

        ii. Concomitantly according to written standard operating procedures which provide for periodic analysis of the test and control articles in the mixture.

B. [Reserved]

C. Where any of the components of the test or control article carrier mixture has an expiration date, that date shall be clearly shown on the container. If more than one component has an expiration date, the earliest date shall be shown.

[43 FR 60013, Dec. 22, 1978, as amended at 45 FR 24865, Apr. 11, 1980; 52 FR 33781, Sept. 4, 1987]

Authority: 21 U.S.C. 342, 346, 346a, 348, 351, 352, 353, 355, 360, 360b-360f, 360h-360j, 371, 379e, 381; 42 U.S.C. 216, 262, 263b-263n.
Source: 43 FR 60013, Dec. 22, 1978, unless otherwise noted.

CHAPTER 8

Subpart G—Protocol for and Conduct of a Nonclinical Laboratory Study
58.120 Protocol.
58.130 Conduct of a nonclinical laboratory study.

Summary

58.120 Protocol—*Each GLP study needs to be conducted according to a study protocol. The process begins with the study director, who writes the study protocol to document what should be done and when as well as anticipated exceptions from SOPs.* Included in the study protocol are descriptions of the experimental design as well as the type and frequency of tests and analyses. The study protocol also documents which records should be archived and available for inspections. Specifically, the study protocol will include:

- Title and statement of the purpose of the study
- Identification of test and control article
- Identification of test system
- Name of the sponsor
- Description of experimental design
- Type and frequency of tests and analyses
- Records to be maintained

58.130 Conduct of a nonclinical laboratory study—In conducting the study, one should strictly follow strictly the protocol, documenting any deviations that may arise. In addition, GLP guidelines also specify how hand-recorded data and data captured from automated equipment should be recorded. For example, hand written data must be recorded in ink and not with a pencil. Changes must not obscure the original entry but and must be dated and signed together with a reason for the change. When data are acquired from an automated system, the person responsible for the system and the system itself should be identified and documented. GLP regulations specify what should be recorded. Examples include:

- Name and address of the laboratory
- Objectives and procedures

-Statistical methods

-Test and control articles, incl. stability data

-Description of methods

-Description of test system

-Description of dosage, route of administration, duration

-Name of the study director

-Location where raw specimens and data are stored

-Descriptions of transformations and calculations (the GLP inspector will want to see how final results have been derived from raw data. So you need to document on paper when you used a calculator, what formulas you have applied in spreadsheets, or what software was used to derive your answers.)

REGULATIONS: Subpart G—Protocol for and Conduct of a Nonclinical Laboratory Study

Sec. 58.120 Protocol.

A. Each study shall have an approved written protocol that clearly indicates the objectives and all methods for the conduct of the study. The protocol shall contain, as applicable, the following information:

1. A descriptive title and statement of the purpose of the study.

2. Identification of the test and control articles by name, chemical abstract number, or code number.

3. The name of the sponsor and the name and address of the testing facility at which the study is being conducted.

4. The number, body weight range, sex, source of supply, species, strain, substrain, and age of the test system.

5. The procedure for identification of the test system.

6. A description of the experimental design, including the methods for the control of bias.

7. A description and/or identification of the diet used in the study as well as solvents, emulsifiers, and/or other materials used to solubilize or suspend the test or control articles before mixing with the carrier. The description shall include specifications for acceptable levels of contaminants that are reasonably expected to be present in the dietary materials and are known to be capable of interfering with the purpose or conduct of the study if present at levels greater than established by the specifications.

8. Each dosage level, expressed in milligrams per kilogram of body weight or other appropriate units, of the test or control article to be administered and the method and frequency of administration.

9. The type and frequency of tests, analyses, and measurements to be made.

10. The records to be maintained.

11. The date of approval of the protocol by the sponsor and the dated signature of the study director.

12. A statement of the proposed statistical methods to be used.

B. All changes in or revisions of an approved protocol and the reasons therefore shall be documented, signed by the study director, dated, and maintained with the protocol.

[43 FR 60013, Dec. 22, 1978, as amended at 52 FR 33781, Sept. 4, 1987; 67 FR 9585, Mar. 4, 2002]

Sec. 58.130 Conduct of a nonclinical laboratory study.

A. The nonclinical laboratory study shall be conducted in accordance with the protocol.

B. The test systems shall be monitored in conformity with the protocol.

C. Specimens shall be identified by test system, study, nature, and date of collection. This information shall be located on the specimen container or shall accompany the specimen in a manner that precludes error in the recording and storage of data.

D. Records of gross findings for a specimen from postmortem observations should be available to a pathologist when examining that specimen histopathologically.

E. All data generated during the conduct of a nonclinical laboratory study, except those that are generated by automated data collection systems, shall be recorded directly, promptly, and legibly in ink. All data entries shall be dated on the date of entry and signed or initialed by the person entering the data. Any change in entries shall be made so as not to obscure the original entry, shall indicate the reason for such change, and shall be dated and signed or identified at the time of the change. In automated data collection systems, the individual responsible for direct data input shall be identified at the time of data input. Any change in automated data entries shall be made so as not to obscure the original entry, shall indicate the reason for change, shall be dated, and the responsible individual shall be identified.

[43 FR 60013, Dec. 22, 1978, as amended at 52 FR 33781, Sept. 4, 1987; 67 FR 9585, Mar. 4, 2002]

Authority: 21 U.S.C. 342, 346, 346a, 348, 351, 352, 353, 355, 360, 360b-360f, 360h-360j, 371, 379e, 381; 42 U.S.C. 216, 262, 263b-263n.
Source: 43 FR 60013, Dec. 22, 1978, unless otherwise noted.

CHAPTER 9

Subpart J—Records and Reports
58.185 Reporting of nonclinical laboratory study results.
58.190 Storage and retrieval of records and data.
58.195 Retention of records.

Summary

58.185 Reporting of nonclinical laboratory study results—This section describes the work up of the final report. Basically, the report is prepared by the laboratory and contains the *what, where, how, and when* of the study. To keep tabs on who was involved, the report is signed and dated by each individual scientist or other professional involved in the study. In addition, to keep track of the data, the report needs to contain the location of where all the specimens, raw data, and the final report are to be stored. When completed, it will need to be run by the quality assurance unit who will review the data, prepare a statement that everything is in order, and sign off on it. Then, and only then, will the report be signed by the study director. Any corrections or additions to a final report need to be in the form of an amendment by the study director. The amendment needs to clearly identify the part of the final report that is being added or corrected, the reasons for these changes, and signatures of those responsible for those changes.

58.190 Storage and retrieval of records and data—These paragraphs basically define *what needs to be retained and how*. Raw data is defined as any laboratory worksheets, records, memoranda, notes, or exact copies thereof, that are the results of original observations and activities of a study. The term covers all data necessary for the reconstruction of the report of the study. Raw data may include hand-written notes, photographs, microfiche copies, computer print-outs, magnetic media, dictated observations, and recorded data from automated instruments. Examples also include records of animal receipt, results of environmental monitoring, instrument calibration records, and integrator output from analytical equipment. Raw data may also be entries in a worksheet used to read and note information from an LED display of an analytical instrument. Raw data are well defined as long as information is recorded on paper. For example original observations are recoded on paper and exact copies can be made if necessary. A more frequently discussed question is what is an exact copy of a paper print-out that comes from an electronic record. Most important here is to look again at the definition of an exact copy: as long as the print-out includes everything that is necessary to reconstruct the study, there should not be a problem. Or as an FDA professional explained to a conference audience: as long as you can demonstrate compliance with the regulation. For example, one requirement of GLP is to document in an audit trail when data have been changed. So look if the print-out includes the audit trail information, for example when data on the computer have been changed. An other question would be if all chromatographic peak in the print-out are on scale? Finally, there should be archives for the orderly storage and quick retrieval of all this data. These archives need to be maintained in such a way to minimize deterioration for the required retention time. This is clearly a lot of work and so GLP requires an archivist. This is either a part time or full time person who is responsible for the archive. Some companies have a procedure that requires documents from an archive to only be checked out by the archivist or his designate. Whenever documents are taken out of the archive this should be documented, and the person who requests it should sign a statement that nothing has been changed, added or deleted. It should be noted that protocols from meetings, if decisions related to the integrity of a study have been made, should also be archived.

58.195 Retention of records--These paragraphs specify how long you'll need to retain your records and specimens. For example, in the US, *material supporting FDA submissions should be retained for 2 years after FDA approval or 5 years after FDA submission.* For wet specimens, the guidelines are more flexible. Basically, wet specimens need only to be retained as long as the quality affords evaluation. Furthermore, this section breaks down how you can store your records. GLP provides the flexibility to either keep the original or an exact copy of a record in the form of a copy from instable thermo paper to durable plain paper or when paper records are scanned into TIF or PDF files. It should be noted that the sponsor company is responsible for the records. When a sponsor company out-sources studies or also just the archiving part, the sponsor company must make sure that archiving of records complies with GLP regulations and in case the contractor goes out of business the sponsor company has access to all data. Finally, make sure to pay special attention to electronic records. Long archiving time as require by GLP typically is no problem for normal paper records, but it may be one for electronic records where software incompatibility issues become a problem. In other words, watch out for those weirdo software programs that go along with things like HPLC data. If you can print them out, then the original can be deleted.

REGULATIONS: Subpart J—Records and Reports

Sec. 58.185 Reporting of nonclinical laboratory study results.

A. A final report shall be prepared for each nonclinical laboratory study and shall include, but not necessarily be limited to, the following:

1. Name and address of the facility performing the study and the dates on which the study was initiated and completed.

2. Objectives and procedures stated in the approved protocol, including any changes in the original protocol.

3. Statistical methods employed for analyzing the data.

4. The test and control articles identified by name, chemical abstracts number or code number, strength, purity, and composition or other appropriate characteristics.

5. Stability of the test and control articles under the conditions of administration.

6. A description of the methods used.

7. A description of the test system used. Where applicable, the final report shall include the number of animals used, sex, body weight range, source of supply, species, strain and substrain, age, and procedure used for identification.

8. A description of the dosage, dosage regimen, route of administration, and duration.

9. A description of all cirmcumstances that may have affected the quality or integrity of the data.

10. The name of the study director, the names of other scientists or professionals, and the names of all supervisory personnel, involved in the study.

11. A description of the transformations, calculations, or operations performed on the data, a summary and analysis of the data, and a statement of the conclusions drawn from the analysis.

12. The signed and dated reports of each of the individual scientists or other professionals involved in the study.

13. The locations where all specimens, raw data, and the final report are to be stored.

14. The statement prepared and signed by the quality assurance unit as described in 58.35(b)(7).

B. The final report shall be signed and dated by the study director.

C. Corrections or additions to a final report shall be in the form of an amendment by the study director. The amendment shall clearly identify that part of the final report that is being added to or corrected and the reasons for the correction or addition, and shall be signed and dated by the person responsible.

[43 FR 60013, Dec. 22, 1978, as amended at 52 FR 33781, Sept. 4, 1987]

Sec. 58.190 Storage and retrieval of records and data.

A. All raw data, documentation, protocols, final reports, and specimens (except those specimens obtained from mutagenicity tests and wet specimens of blood, urine, feces, and biological fluids) generated as a result of a nonclinical laboratory study shall be retained.

B. There shall be archives for orderly storage and expedient retrieval of all raw data, documentation, protocols, specimens, and interim and final reports. Conditions of storage shall minimize deterioration of the documents or specimens in accordance with the requirements for the time period of their retention and the nature of the documents or specimens. A testing facility may contract with commercial archives to provide a repository for all material to be retained. Raw data and specimens may be retained elsewhere provided that the archives have specific reference to those other locations.

C. An individual shall be identified as responsible for the archives.

D. Only authorized personnel shall enter the archives.

E. Material retained or referred to in the archives shall be indexed to permit expedient retrieval.

[43 FR 60013, Dec. 22, 1978, as amended at 52 FR 33781, Sept. 4, 1987; 67 FR 9585, Mar. 4, 2002]

Sec. 58.195 Retention of records.

A. Record retention requirements set forth in this section do not supersede the record retention requirements of any other regulations in this chapter.

B. Except as provided in paragraph (c) of this section, documentation records, raw data and specimens pertaining to a nonclinical laboratory study and required to be made by this part shall be retained in the archive(s) for whichever of the following periods is shortest:

1. A period of at least 2 years following the date on which an application for a research or marketing permit, in support of which the results of the nonclinical laboratory study were submitted, is approved by the Food and Drug Administration. This requirement does not apply to studies supporting investigational new drug applications (IND's) or applications for investigational device exemptions (IDE's), records of which shall be governed by the provisions of paragraph (b)(2) of this section.

2. A period of at least 5 years following the date on which the results of the nonclinical laboratory study are submitted to the Food and Drug Administration in support of an application for a research or marketing permit.

3. In other situations (e.g., where the nonclinical laboratory study does not result in the submission of the study in support of an application for a research or marketing permit), a period of at least 2 years following the date on which the study is completed, terminated, or discontinued.

C. Wet specimens (except those specimens obtained from mutagenicity tests and wet specimens of blood, urine, feces, and biological fluids), samples of test or control articles, and specially prepared material, which are relatively fragile and differ markedly in stability and quality during storage, shall be retained only as long as the quality of the preparation affords evaluation. In no case shall retention be required for longer periods than those set forth in paragraphs (a) and (b) of this section.

D. The master schedule sheet, copies of protocols, and records of quality assurance inspections, as required by 58.35(c) shall be maintained by the quality assurance unit as an easily accessible system of records for the period of time specified in paragraphs (a) and (b) of this section.

E. Summaries of training and experience and job descriptions required to be maintained by 58.29(b) may be retained along with all other testing facility employment records for the length of time specified in paragraphs (a) and (b) of this section.

F. Records and reports of the maintenance and calibration and inspection of equipment, as required by 58.63(b) and (c), shall be retained for the length of time specified in paragraph (b) of this section.

G. Records required by this part may be retained either as original records or as true copies such as photocopies, microfilm, microfiche, or other accurate reproductions of the original records.

H. If a facility conducting nonclinical testing goes out of business, all raw data, documentation, and other material specified in this section shall be transferred to the archives of the sponsor of the study. The Food and Drug Administration shall be notified in writing of such a transfer.

[43 FR 60013, Dec. 22, 1978, as amended at 52 FR 33781, Sept. 4, 1987; 54 FR 9039, Mar. 3, 1989]

Authority: 21 U.S.C. 342, 346, 346a, 348, 351, 352, 353, 355, 360, 360b-360f, 360h-360j, 371, 379e, 381; 42 U.S.C. 216, 262, 263b-263n.
Source: 43 FR 60013, Dec. 22, 1978, unless otherwise noted.

CHAPTER 10

Subpart K— Disqualification of Testing Facilities

58.200 Purpose.

58.202 Grounds for disqualification.

58.204 Notice of and opportunity for hearing on proposed disqualification.

58.206 Final order on disqualification.

58.210 Actions upon disqualification.

58.213 Public disclosure of information regarding disqualification.

58.215 Alternative or additional actions to disqualification.

58.217 Suspension or termination of a testing facility by a sponsor.

58.219 Reinstatement of a disqualified testing facility.

Summary

Basically, this entire subpart describes how you can get your study disqualified, the legal route of disqualification, your rights to challenge disqualification, and route to reinstatement following a disqualification. However, rather than mull on the negatives, lets go over what the FDA wants to see, why, when, and what happens if you're not in compliance:

It is FDA's responsibility to enforce the federal Food, drug and Cosmetic Act to ensure safety and effectiveness of drugs and medical devices. This is enforced through regulations, guidance documents and FDA inspections. The FDA has the responsibility to inspect GLP studies related to products that are marketed in the United States. So basically, it doesn't mattered where the products are developed or manufactured.

The inspection program the FDA has developed falls into two types:

-Routine inspection

-For cause inspection

Routine inspections should be conducted at least every second year. It is an on-going evaluation of a laboratory's compliance with GLP regulation. For cause inspections are less frequent, they constitute only about 20% of all GLP inspections. Reasons for such inspections could be a follow up of an inspection with serious deficiencies or when the FDA suspect non-compliance when investigating NDA applications. It also may happen that the FDA gets some hints from external sources about non-compliance in laboratories. Typically the FDA does not announce GLP inspections. If a laboratory refuses to accept FDA inspections, either in full or also part of it, the FDA will not accept studies in support of new drug applications.

Deviations from GLP requirements are documented in different ways: if the inspection team finds deviations, they write them in a specific form which has the number 483. The deviations are discussed during the exit meeting and the laboratory can respond. Then the lead inspector writes a full inspection report which is called the *establishment inspection report*. This may be up to 20 or 30 pages. Depending on the deviations the inspector will or will not to write a warning letter. This letter is sent to the company's management. Within 14 days the company needs to respond with a corrective action plan or risk the disqualification of their study.

REGULATIONS: Subpart K— Disqualification of Testing Facilities

Sec. 58.200 Purpose.

A. The purposes of disqualification are:

1. To permit the exclusion from consideration of completed studies that were conducted by a testing facility which has failed to comply with the requirements of the good laboratory practice regulations until it can be adequately demonstrated that such noncompliance did not occur during, or did not affect the validity or acceptability of data generated by, a particular study; and

2. To exclude from consideration all studies completed after the date of disqualification until the facility can satisfy the Commissioner that it will conduct studies in compliance with such regulations.

B. The determination that a nonclinical laboratory study may not be considered in support of an application for a research or marketing permit does not, however, relieve the applicant for such a permit of any obligation under any other applicable regulation to submit the results of the study to the Food and Drug Administration.

Sec. 58.202 Grounds for disqualification.

The Commissioner may disqualify a testing facility upon finding all of the following:

A. The testing facility failed to comply with one or more of the regulations set forth in this part (or any other regulations regarding such facilities in this chapter);

B. The noncompliance adversely affected the validity of the nonclinical laboratory studies; and

C. Other lesser regulatory actions (e.g., warnings or rejection of individual studies) have not been or will probably not be adequate to achieve compliance with the good laboratory practice regulations.

Sec. 58.204 Notice of and opportunity for hearing on proposed disqualification.

A. Whenever the Commissioner has information indicating that grounds exist under 58.202 which in his opinion justify disqualification of a testing facility, he may issue to the testing facility a written notice proposing that the facility be disqualified.

B. A hearing on the disqualification shall be conducted in accordance with the requirements for a regulatory hearing set forth in part 16 of this chapter.

Sec. 58.206 Final order on disqualification.

A. If the Commissioner, after the regulatory hearing, or after the time for requesting a hearing expires without a request being made, upon an evaulation of the administrative record of the disqualification proceeding, makes the findings required in 58.202, he shall issue a final order disqualifying the facility. Such order shall include a statement of the basis for that determination. Upon issuing a final order, the Commissioner shall notify (with a copy of the order) the testing facility of the action.

B. If the Commissioner, after a regulatory hearing or after the time for requesting a hearing expires without a request being made, upon an evaluation of the administrative record of the disqualification proceeding, does not make the findings required in 58.202, he shall issue a final order terminating the disqualification proceeding. Such order shall include a statement of the basis for that determination. Upon issuing a final order the Commissioner shall notify the testing facility and provide a copy of the order.

Sec. 58.210 Actions upon disqualification.

A. Once a testing facility has been disqualified, each application for a research or marketing permit, whether approved or not, containing or relying upon any nonclinical laboratory study conducted by the disqualified testing facility may be examined to determine whether such study was or would be essential to a decision. If it is determined that a study was or would be essential, the Food and Drug Administration shall also determine whether the study is acceptable, notwithstanding the disqualification of the facility. Any study done by a testing facility before or after disqualification may be presumed to be unacceptable, and the person relying on the study may be required to establish that the study was not affected by the circumstances that led to the disqualification, e.g., by submitting validating information. If the study is then determined to be unacceptable, such data will be eliminated from consideration in support of the application; and such elimination may serve as new information justifying the termination or withdrawal of approval of the application.

B. No nonclinical laboratory study begun by a testing facility after the date of the facility's disqualification shall be considered in support of any application for a research or marketing permit, unless the facility has been reinstated under 58.219. The determination that a study may not be considered in support of an application for a research or marketing permit does not, however, relieve the applicant for such a permit of any obligation under any other applicable regulation to submit the results of the study to the Food and Drug Administration.

[43 FR 60013, Dec. 22, 1978, as amended at 59 FR 13200, Mar. 21, 1994]

Sec. 58.213 Public disclosure of information regarding disqualification.

A. Upon issuance of a final order disqualifying a testing facility under 58.206(a), the Commissioner may notify all or any interested persons. Such notice may be given at the discretion of the Commissioner whenever he believes that such disclosure would further the public interest or would promote compliance with the good laboratory practice regulations set forth in this part. Such notice, if given, shall include a copy of the final order issued under 58.206(a) and shall state that the disqualification constitutes a determination by the Food and Drug Administration that nonclinical laboratory studies performed by the facility will not be considered by the Food and Drug Administration in support of any application for a research or marketing permit. If such notice is sent to another Federal Government agency, the Food and Drug Administration will recommend that the agency also consider whether or not it should accept nonclinical laboratory studies performed by the testing facility. If such notice is sent to any other person, it shall state that it is given because of the relationship between the testing facility and the person being notified and that the Food and Drug Administration is not advising or recommending that any action be taken by the person notified.

B. A determination that a testing facility has been disqualified and the administrative record regarding such determination are disclosable to the public under part 20 of this chapter.

Sec. 58.215 Alternative or additional actions to disqualification.

A. Disqualification of a testing facility under this subpart is independent of, and neither in lieu of nor a precondition to, other proceedings or actions authorized by the act. The Food and Drug Administration may, at any time, institute against a testing facility and/or against the sponsor of a nonclinical laboratory study that has been submitted to the Food and Drug Administration any appropriate judicial proceedings (civil or criminal) and any other appropriate regulatory action, in addition to or in lieu of, and prior to, simultaneously with, or subsequent to, disqualification. The Food and Drug

Administration may also refer the matter to another Federal, State, or local government law enforcement or regulatory agency for such action as that agency deems appropriate.

B. The Food and Drug Administration may refuse to consider any particular nonclinical laboratory study in support of an application for a research or marketing permit, if it finds that the study was not conducted in accordance with the good laboratory practice regulations set forth in this part, without disqualifying the testing facility that conducted the study or undertaking other regulatory action.

Sec. 58.217 Suspension or termination of a testing facility by a sponsor.

Termination of a testing facility by a sponsor is independent of, and neither in lieu of nor a precondition to, proceedings or actions authorized by this subpart. If a sponsor terminates or suspends a testing facility from further participation in a nonclinical laboratory study that is being conducted as part of any application for a research or marketing permit that has been submitted to any Center of the Food and Drug Administration (whether approved or not), it shall notify that Center in writing within 15 working days of the action; the notice shall include a statement of the reasons for such action. Suspension or termination of a testing facility by a sponsor does not relieve it of any obligation under any other applicable regulation to submit the results of the study to the Food and Drug Administration.

[43 FR FR 60013, Dec. 22, 1978, as amended at 50 FR 8995, Mar. 6, 1985]

Sec. 58.219 Reinstatement of a disqualified testing facility.

A testing facility that has been disqualified may be reinstated as an acceptable source of nonclinical laboratory studies to be submitted to the Food and Drug Administration if the Commissioner determines, upon an evaluation of the submission of the testing facility, that the facility can adequately assure that it will conduct future nonclinical laboratory studies in compliance with the good laboratory practice regulations set forth in this part and, if any studies are currently being conducted, that the quality and integrity of such studies have not been seriously compromised. A disqualified testing facility that wishes to be so reinstated shall present in writing to the Commissioner reasons why it believes it should be reinstated and a detailed description of the corrective actions it has taken or intends to take to assure that the acts or omissions which led to its disqualification will not recur. The Commissioner may condition reinstatement upon the testing facility being found in compliance with the good laboratory practice regulations upon an inspection. If a testing facility is reinstated, the Commissioner shall so notify the testing facility and all organizations and persons who were notified, under 58.213 of the disqualification of the testing facility. A determination that a testing facility has been reinstated is disclosable to the public under part 20 of this chapter.

Authority: 21 U.S.C. 342, 346, 346a, 348, 351, 352, 353, 355, 360, 360b-360f, 360h-360j, 371, 379e, 381; 42 U.S.C. 216, 262, 263b-263n.
Source: 43 FR 60013, Dec. 22, 1978, unless otherwise noted.